I0419626

SIMPLY SATISFYING

7 Days of Simple Meals With Extra Room For Treats

. . . .

BY: KATIE TEDDER

Keep in Mind:

Every Body is different, so the plans that I'm about to share with you are a general healthy breakdown of macronutrients (carbohydrates, proteins, and fats) that would benefit most women to some degree.   However, calorie range, goals, body type, and activity level all play a part in what your daily meals should look like. These meals should be adjusted accordingly to what is specific to you and your needs and goals. One take away that I would like you to get from this meal plan booklet is that it is possible to live a healthy lifestyle and reach your goals, while still enjoying things you love.

Why 1400 Calorie Meal Plans?

If you weigh at least 140 pounds and your goal is to lose weight, then this book will benefit you as written. All the plans in this book are formulated to a 1400 calorie target goal, because it is a good target number for a wide variety of women. With that said, there are some tips you can follow to adjust it to fit your needs better.

* If you weigh less than 140 lbs and still want to lose weight, you can easily cut out 100-200 calories by cutting out one snack option in each day. This will bring the plan from 1400 down to 1200-1300 calories. You'll learn that little tweaks like this can make a big difference.

* If you find that you are losing weight too quickly, (a healthy weight loss is 1-2 lbs per week) you can start with doubling a snack option. Not the desserts...we are working on moderation, not excuses to indulge. This could take your plan to 1500-1600, which might be a better fit for you.

Helpful Tips Before You Start:

❖ **Rearrange If You Need To:**

Rearrange the meals around, within the day in which you are following, to make it fit better for your schedule. If you need to combine a snack with lunch, that's okay! The goal is to finish eating everything on the list by the end of the day.

❖ **Substitute With Similar Foods:**

If you do not like an item on the menu, try to replace it with a similar one. For example: If you don't like carrots, pick another vegetable. If you don't like Pork Chops…pick another meat/fish.

❖ **Save Room For The Reward:**

Remember, in order to enjoy the treats you really want to eat, adjustments have to be made during the other meals. This means that you need to follow the portion sizes with your other meals in order to have room for your dessert. A couple extra bites here and a couple extra bites there will add up to equal or surpass the allotment you saved for your treat. Just remember, THERE IS A REWARD AT THE END OF THE DAY YOU WANT TO ENJOY! There is no need to indulge all day!

❖ The Goal Is To Eventually Choose Healthier Alternatives:

The purpose of this book is to open your eyes to a healthy and balanced lifestyle at any level. As you continue your health journey, you will be ready to find healthier replacements for these treats that will satisfy you just as much. Then, maybe one day you won't even need the treats. But for now, eat healthy and balanced and still enjoy your treat.

GROCERY LIST

....

CARBOHYDRATES

- Whole Wheat Bread
- Whole Wheat Buns
- Whole Wheat Tortillas
- Taco Shells
- Waffles (frozen)
- Pancake Mix
- Potatoes
- Spaghetti
- Brown Rice
- Raisin Bran Cereal (or something similar)
- Baked Beans
- Mixed Greens
- Spinach
- Cucumbers
- Baby Carrots
- Broccoli
- Bell Peppers
- Onions
- Tomatoes
- Celery
- Pasta Sauce
- Fat Free Sour Cream
- Taco Seasoning
- Vegetable Soup or Chicken/ Beef Broth
- Medium Sized Apples
- Bananas
- Small Oranges
- Frozen Mangos
- Frozen Blueberries
- Frozen and Fresh Strawberries
- Milk
- Tri Zero Oikos Yogurt (Choose your Flavor)
- Chocolate Chip Cookie Dough
- Wine (red or white)
- Milk Duds or Fun Sized M&Ms
- Hershey Syrup
- Waffle Cones
- Vanilla or Chocolate Ice Cream
- Brownie Mix
- Dark Chocolate Chips (at least 60% cocoa)
- Potato Chip Snack Packs

GROCERY LIST

PROTEINS

- Eggs
- Turkey Sausage
- Turkey Bacon
- Boneless Pork Chops
- Lunch Meat Ham
- Ground Beef 95% lean
- Salmon
- Chicken Tenderloins
- Beef Chuck for Stew

- Protein Powder. (look for higher grams of protein and lower grams of carbohydrates)

FATS

- Butter
- Almond Milk
- Turkey Bacon
- Lite Balsamic Vinaigrette
- Shredded Cheese
- Peanut Butter/Almond Butter
- Nutella
- Extra Virgin Olive Oil
- Cheese Slices (you pick)
- Trail Mix
- Pesto Sauce

MONDAY
Save Room For That Cookie!

BREAKFAST

1 Whole Egg
1/2 Slice of Whole Wheat Buttered Toast
2 Turkey Sausage Links
Enjoy a cup of coffee or tea!

SNACK

1 Scoop of your choice of Protein Powder
8 oz Almond Milk (or water)
1/2 Frozen Banana
Blend Together And Enjoy!

LUNCH

1-2 Grilled Chicken Tenderloins
1 c. Spinach along with any other veggie you enjoy
1 Tbsp Balsamic Vinaigrette Lite Dressing
Enjoy your grilled chicken wrap.

SNACK

1 Handful of baby carrots
1 Small orange

DINNER

1 Boneless Pork Chop
(not breaded...season with salt and pepper)
1 Medium Potato (you can do 1 serving of mashed also)
1 cup of your favorite veggie

SNACK

2 Chocolate Chip Cookies
4 oz Glass of milk if you'd like to dip

1400 Calorie Per Day Plan.
Balanced Macros of 40% Carbs. 30% Protein. 30%Fats

NOT FEELING
CHOCOLATE CHIP COOKIES?

That's okay!
2 chocolate chip cookies with milk equals about
320 calories all together.

You may have to look at some labels, but I'm sure you can
find something in your house that you enjoy for 320
calories.

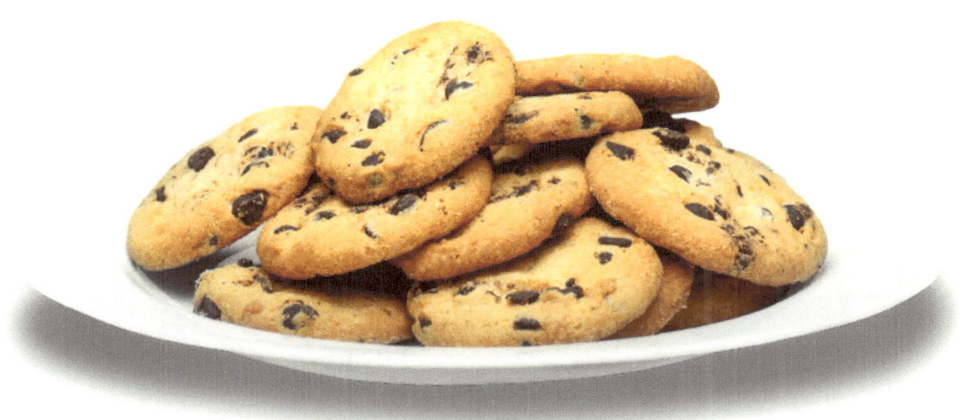

TUESDAY
Save Room For That Ice Cream!

BREAKFAST
1 Waffle
Don't use syrup. Instead heat up 1/2 c. Frozen Blueberries, mix with a sprinkle of sugar and top your waffle with that mixture.
Enjoy a cup of coffee or tea!

SNACK
1 Scoop of your favorite Protein Powder
8 oz Water
1 c. Frozen Strawberries
Blend and Enjoy!

LUNCH
3oz Grilled Chicken tenderloins
1 c. Spinach
1/2 c. Mixed Greens
Cucumbers and Carrots
1 tbsp Balsamic Vinaigrette
Enjoy your Salad!

SNACK
Sorry, no snack today!
You want ice cream later, remember?

DINNER
1 Beef Patty on a Whole Wheat Bun
Topped with a Slice of Cheese
Lettuce, Tomato, and Onion and ketchup and Mustard
1/4 c. Baked Beans

SNACK
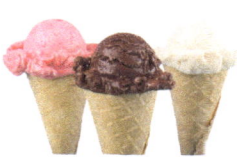
1/2 cup Haagen-Dazs Ice Cream (choc. or vanilla)
OR
You can have 1 cup of Breyer's Ice Cream
(choc. or vanilla)
Waffle Cone (from a store...not ice cream shop)

1400 Calorie Per Day Plan.
Balanced Macros of 40% Carbs. 30% Protein. 30%Fats

NOT DIGGING ICE CREAM TONIGHT?

That's okay!
A 1/2c. Haagen-Dazs Ice Cream with a waffle cone
drizzled with chocolate syrup is around 380 calories.

You can decrease this calorie amount by about 100
calories by just choosing a different brand of ice cream.

If you want your ice cream in a bowl, you can drizzle a
little more chocolate on top or drizzle a tbsp of
peanut butter on top.

You may have to look at some labels, but I'm sure you can
find a replacement for less than 380 calories.

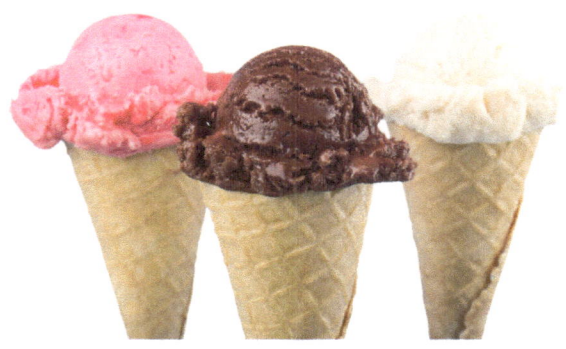

WEDNESDAY
Save Room For That Brownie!

BREAKFAST
3 Egg Whites
2 Turkey Sausage Links
Enjoy a cup of coffee or tea!

SNACK
1 Scoop of Your Favorite Protein Powder
8oz Water
1 c. Frozen Blueberries
Blend and Enjoy!

LUNCH
1/2 Ham Sandwich using 1 slice of Whole Wheat Bread
1 Slice of Cheese
Lettuce and Mustard
1 handful of Veggie Sticks on the side.

SNACK
23 Almonds or Mixed Nuts
(You can also swap these nuts for the veggies and enjoy the nuts for lunch instead.)

DINNER
Beef Stew in the Crock Pot
Prepare in the Morning.
Add Beef, Potatoes, Carrots, Celery, Diced Tomatoes, Beef Broth,
Seasonings You Like, and Water
Enjoy a big bowl of it!

SNACK
1 Brownie with 4 oz of milk

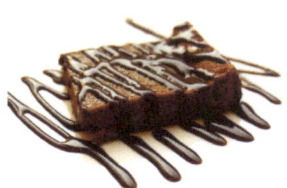

1400 Calorie Per Day Plan.
Balanced Macros of 40% Carbs. 30% Protein. 30%Fats

NOT FEELING THE BROWNIE?

That's okay!
1 Brownie with 4oz of Milk equals around 135 calories.

You may have to look at some labels, but I'm sure you can find something you enjoy for 135 calories.
Make sure not to go over!

We are enjoying treats in moderation!

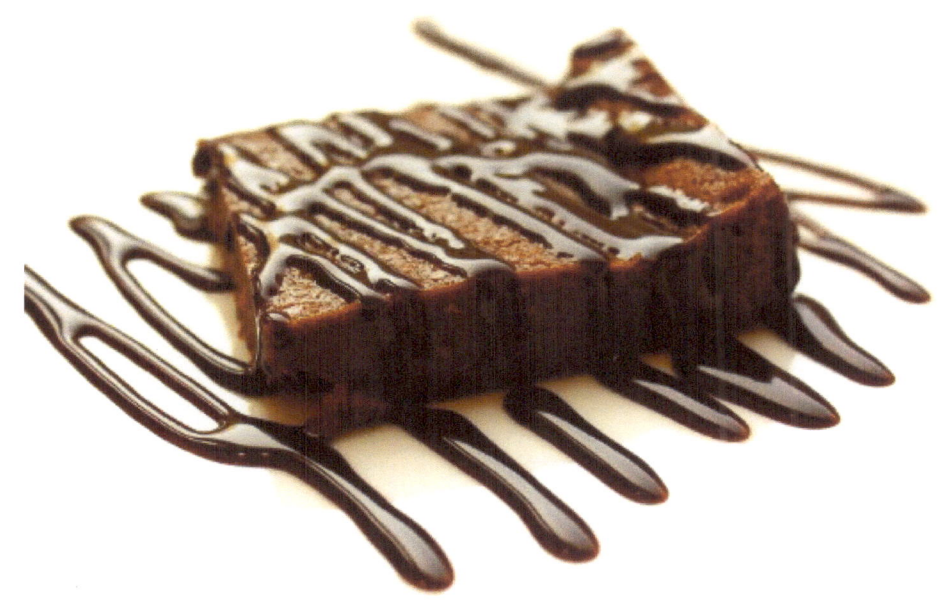

THURSDAY
Save Room For Some Candy Treats!

BREAKFAST
1 Serving of Raisin Bran Cereal
Or A Similar Cereal...no sugary sugar puffs!
Add Milk
Enjoy a cup of coffee or tea!

SNACK
1 Scoop of Your Favorite Protein Powder
8oz Almond Milk
1/2 Frozen Banana
2 tbsp Almond Butter
Blend and Enjoy!
If you don't have a blender, Shake the Powder and Milk together and enjoy your banana and peanut butter separately.

LUNCH
1 Bowl Chicken & Vegetable Soup
Homemade or Canned

SNACK
1 Tri Zero Oikos Yogurt ANY FLAVOR
(I like this brand because it has a higher protein content than other yogurts)

DINNER
1 Salmon Fillet Seasoned and Baked
1/2 c. Brown Rice
1 c. Steamed Broccoli

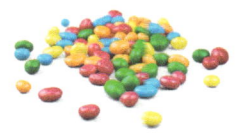

SNACK
2 Fun Size Boxes/Bags of Candy

1400 Calorie Per Day Plan.
Balanced Macros of 40% Carbs. 30% Protein. 30%Fats

NOT IN THE MOOD FOR CANDY TONIGHT?

That's okay!
2 fun size boxes of Milk Duds equals 104 calories.

2 fun sized bags of m&ms equals 146 calories.

Whatever you eat, you Do Not want to go over 150 calories.

2 Oreo Cookies is 106 calories.

2 cups of Microwaved Popcorn is 128 calories.

We are enjoying treats in moderation!

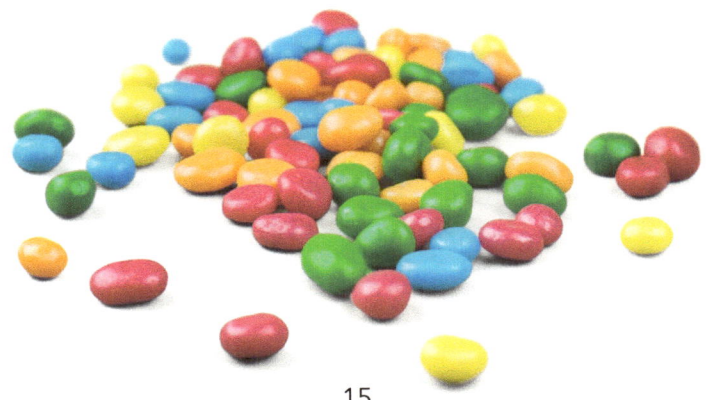

FRIDAY
Enjoy A Glass Of Wine Today!

BREAKFAST
Egg White Omelet:
Use 4 Egg Whites (no yolk)
Sauté 1 c. of your favorite veggies and
1 Slice chopped Ham for your omelet filling
Top with 2 tbsp Shredded Cheese
Enjoy your coffee or tea!

SNACK
8 oz Water
1/2 c. Frozen Mangos
1 Scoop Protein Powder
Blend and Enjoy

LUNCH
1/2 BLT Sandwich:
2 Halves Whole Wheat Bread
3 Slices Turkey Bacon
Lettuce and Slices of Tomato
With a side:
1 individual container of Tri Zero Oikos Yogurt

SNACK
1 Medium Apple Sliced
Dip in 1 Tbsp Peanut Butter or Almond Butter

DINNER
Spaghetti With Ground Meat Sauce:
1/2 c. Spaghetti Pasta
3 oz Ground Beef (seasoned)
1 c. Spaghetti Sauce (jarred or homemade)
Use 1 tbsp Olive oil for cooking
Make yourself a bowl of side salad to go with it.

SNACK
5 oz Glass of Wine (red or white)

1400 Calorie Per Day Plan.
Balanced Macros of 40% Carbs. 30% Protein. 30%Fats

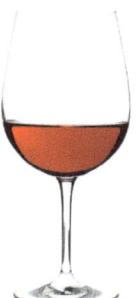

NOT A BIG DRINKER?

That's okay!
A 5 oz glass of wine is around 150 calories.

You may have to look at some labels, but I'm sure you can find something in your house that you enjoy for 150 calories.

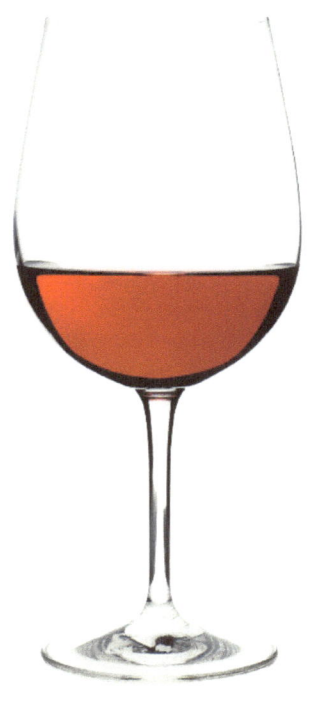

SATURDAY
Save Room For Chips!

BREAKFAST
2 four inch Pancakes
Top with 1/2 c. Frozen Blueberries or Strawberries
(heated in microwave and mix with a sprinkle of sugar)
1 Fried Egg White as a side

SNACK
Strawberry Chip Shake:
8oz Water
1/2 c. Frozen Strawberries
1 Scoop Protein Powder
16 Dark Chocolate Chips
Blend and Enjoy!

LUNCH
Grilled Chicken Salad:
4oz Grilled Chicken
1 Handful of Mixed Greens
Top with 1 c. of your favorite veggies
1 tbsp Lite Balsamic Vinaigrette

SNACK
1 Snack Pack of Trail Mix

DINNER
Chicken Pesto Pizza:
1 Whole Wheat Tortilla
Lightly Spread Pesto Sauce
Layer with a lot of veggies, tomatoes, and spinach
Top with 2 oz Shredded Chicken
Sprinkle 1/4 c. Shredded Mozzarella
Bake in the oven at 375 for 6-8 minutes.
*Cooking time will depend on the thickness of the toppings.

SNACK
1 Snack Bag of Potato Chips or something similar

1400 Calorie Per Day Plan.
Balanced Macros of 40% Carbs. 30% Protein. 30%Fats

NOT IN THE MOOD FOR POTATO CHIPS?

That's okay!
A snack bag of potato chips is around 150 calories.

You may have to look at some labels, but I'm sure you can find something in your house that you enjoy for
150 calories.

Don't forget to look back at the other days in this book. Some of the other dessert options could be inserted into this day as well.

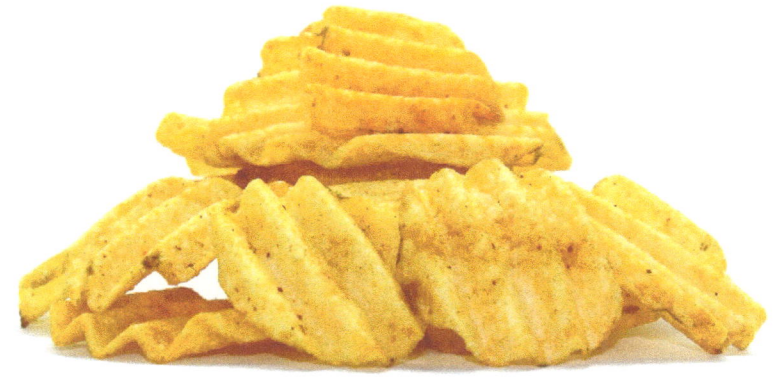

SUNDAY
Save Room For Nutella!

BREAKFAST
1 Egg White
3 Slices of Turkey Bacon
1/2 slice of Whole Wheat Toast, light on the Butter.

SNACK
8 oz Almond Milk
1 Scoop of your favorite Protein Powder

LUNCH
1/2 Ham Sandwich:
1 Slice of Whole Wheat Bread
Ham lunchmeat. You can use Turkey too.
Top with Lettuce, Tomato, and Onions if you'd like.
Use mustard. Avoid Mayo.

1 individual container of Tri Zero Oikos Yogurt

SNACK
4 Celery Sticks
6 Baby Carrots
1 tbsp Hummus (can be the flavored kind)

DINNER
Tacos

3 oz Ground Beef with taco seasoning
2 Hard Taco Shells (or 2 small soft shells)
2 Tbsp of Sour Cream (1 in each shell)
2 Tbsp of Salsa (1 in each shell)
1/4 c. Shredded Cheese (split between 2 tacos)
1 c. Shredded Lettuce (split between two tacos)

SNACK
2 Tbsp Nutella
1 c. of Fresh Strawberries
You can heat the Nutella slightly and drizzle it over the strawberries.

1400 Calorie Per Day Plan.
Balanced Macros of 40% Carbs. 30% Protein. 30%Fats

NOT IN THE MOOD FOR NUTELLA?

That's okay!
2 Tbsp of Nutella and 1 c. of Strawberries is around
250 calories.

If you have had your fill for desserts this week and don't
really want a treat, plan ahead and add the 1c. of fruit and
2 tbsp peanut butter to your protein shake instead.

If you're still enjoying all the treats you've been allowed
to have, don't forget to look at your labels and find
something worth 250 calories.

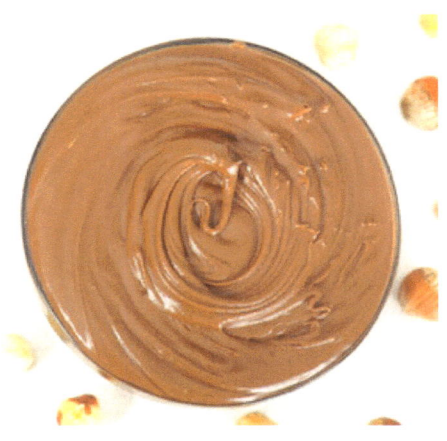

100-200 calorie
Healthy Treat & Snack Ideas:

Though you may be enjoying your treats...the goal is to eventually find healthier alternatives to replace those sweet cravings. Below is a list of healthier treat options that you can try instead to fit into your meals:

* 1/2 Apple with 1 tbsp Peanut Butter
* 100 calorie bags of Popcorn
* 10 Baked Tortilla Chips with 1/2 c. salsa
* 1 Apple and 1 String Cheese
* 1/2 English Muffin with 2 Tbsp Cream Cheese
* 1/4 c. Almonds, Pistachios, or Cashews
* 1/2 c. Frozen Yogurt
* 1/2 c. Cottage Cheese with Mandarin Oranges
* 1/2 c. Sorbet or Sherbet
* 2 Large Hard Boil Eggs
* 100 Calorie Snack Packs

Thank You

I hope you enjoyed this book. This is just a glimpse into my individualized nutrition coaching. This is what I do! I take foods that you love to eat and try to work them in appropriately to your day, so you can still work towards your goals without getting frustrated with recipes that are unrealistic on a daily basis.

I also help you choose healthier versions of foods that really aren't good for you. It's all about finding the right balance that works for you specifically, so you can be consistent. Consistency will show results.

If you are interested in more specific daily plans that will help you reach your own personal goals, feel free to contact me at katy@katydidfitness.com or check out my website, https://katydidfitness.com.

You can also follow me on Facebook, Pinterest, Instagram, and Twitter. Just search Katydid Fitness.

I'd be happy to help you work towards your goals!

Katie Tedder

Your Personal Notes:

Your Personal Notes:

www.ingramcontent.com/pod-procuct-compliance
Lightning Source LLC
Chambersburg PA
CBHW060824290526

45792CB00005BB/1792